Intermittent Fasting:

Ultimate Beginner's Guide to Simple Weight Loss, Fat Burn and A Healthy Body

Jamie Connor

purview. There are no scenarios in which the publisher or the original author of this work can be in any fashion deemed liable for any hardship or damages that may befall them after undertaking information described herein.

Additionally, the information in the following pages is intended only for informational purposes and should thus be thought of as universal. As befitting its nature, it is presented without assurance regarding its prolonged validity or interim quality. Trademarks that are mentioned are done without written consent and can in no way be considered an endorsement from the trademark holder.

Table of Contents

Introduction

Congratulations on downloading **Intermittent Fasting: Ultimate Guide to Simple Weight Loss, Fat Burn and a Healthy Body** and thank you for doing so.

The following chapters will discuss what is intermittent fasting, what types of protocols it involves, the benefits of such a lifestyle and how to make it part of your life. There has been a lot of interest and research into intermittent fasting and the benefits it has.

Many people who want to stay healthy, fit, avoid chronic illnesses and live longer are choosing intermittent fasting as a way of life as it is a great way to achieve a healthier, leaner body in no time. The best thing about intermittent fasting is that you can choose what you want to eat. The protocol only dictates *when* to eat. Calories can also be restricted to promote weight loss.

There are plenty of books on this subject on the market, thanks again for choosing this one! Every effort was made to ensure it is full of as much useful information as possible. Please enjoy!

Chapter 1: What is Intermittent Fasting?

A new and exciting phenomenon known as *intermittent fasting* is now one of the most popular health and fitness trends in the world. This phenomenon is considered more of a lifestyle than a diet or temporary trend. But what exactly is intermittent fasting and how do you go about it?

Defining Intermittent Fasting

Intermittent fasting can be defined as an eating pattern that consists of two distinct periods of fasting and eating. Numerous studies show that alternating cycles of fasting and eating can result in weight loss, better metabolism, and numerous other health benefits.

It involves making a conscious decision to deliberately skip some meals and eat later. This lifestyle simply implies that you only take in calories at a specific time of the day and then not consume any food for the remaining part of the day. Intermittent fasting is more than just a diet. It is a lifestyle that alternates between periods of fasting and non-fasting.

The Origins of Fasting

The term fasting refers to the deliberate abstinence from food, drink, or both for a limited period of time. There are different types of fasting practiced around the world. Absolute fasting, for instance, means complete abstinence from all food and drink for a definite period of time, often for a period of 24 hours.

Fasting has been practiced by man since ancient times. It is a natural recourse for humans and animals to fast during times of illness or stress. Fasting provides balance, rest, and helps to conserve energy at critical times. Early philosophers, great thinkers, and healers used fasting as a healing therapy for health purposes. Records have shown that Hippocrates who was the father of modern medicine said "eating while being sick, is to feed the sickness". Plutarch who was a Greek philosopher said "Instead of using medicine, rather, fast a day". Other famous philosophers and great thinkers include Socrates, Plato, Aristotle, and Galen.

Fasting is still common to most religions including Christianity, Islam, and Buddhism. Indians from both North and South America have been known to fast as part of their traditions. Yoga practice, which includes elements of fasting, has been around for thousands of years. To this very day, the ancient healing practices of Ayurveda also include fasting as a form of therapy.

Fasting in the 19th Century

Intermittent fasting was first tried by health experts in the early 1900s to treat different disorders like obesity, epilepsy, and diabetes. It is now making a comeback and is proving popular among different groups in society. It is popular mostly with people who wish to lose weight.

Intermittent fasting is not new to humans. We have been fasting for a long time, especially the typical overnight fast. However, doctors recently started clinical research on the benefits of intermittent fasting on longevity and overall health. It is these findings that have caught the eye of health enthusiasts and people all around the world. Many are of the view that intermittent fasting is a lifestyle we have been looking for and not one that we are forced to endure.

Reasons why People Fast

There are many reasons why people fast. According to Paracelsus, the father of modern medicine, fasting is the greatest remedy and the physician within. It is said that fasting has been recognized as a mode of caring for the sick. Here are reasons why people choose to fast.

Medical reasons –diagnostic purposes, medical procedure

Health reasons – Retuning the body

Religious reasons – spiritual enlightenment

Political reasons – standing up for a cause

Why Intermittent Fasting is popular among Women

One of the main reasons why women choose intermittent fasting over other weight loss diets or lifestyles is that they can lose weight and keep it off. It provides an excellent pathway of getting rid of stubborn tummy fat and excessive body weight.

Intermittent fasting does not demand adherence to any challenging diet or calorie restrictions. It, instead, provides one of the easiest ways of losing the bad weight while maintaining good fat and muscle. There is no requirement to change eating habits. A lot of women have successfully adopted this lifestyle for several reasons such as losing their baby weight and regaining control over crazy eating habits.

A Lifestyle Rather Than a Diet

Intermittent fasting is seen more as a way of life rather than a diet. There is nothing about which foods you should eat but, rather, when you should eat. There are different protocols of this kind of fasting with each protocol splitting a day or week into eating and fasting periods.

Many people have taken to intermittent fasting and turned it into a lifestyle. Think about having a switch that can balance your metabolism and perform a deep cleanse without using costly detoxification kits. The body has an excellent mechanism that can achieve this. This mechanism is known autophagy, and it is simply another term for intermittent fasting.

What is Autophagy?

It is your body's ultimate recycling system. Autophagy replaces damaged and worn-out parts of your cells with new ones, thereby helping to preserve tissue health. The cells in your body create membranes that hunt down diseased, dead, and worn-out cells and then consumes them, using the resulting molecules to make new cell parts and for energy. In the process, the cells also consume harmful organisms such as disease-causing bacteria.

Thus old and worn-out bits are consumed by the cells within your body which creates fuel as well as parts for new cells. Cells in your body sometimes digest proteins to release amino acids and provide much-needed energy. This process, known as autophagy, is essential as it promotes metabolism and slows down the aging process.

Celebrities and Intermittent Fasting

A lot of well-known celebrities have also turned to intermittent fasting lately. They have turned to this form of lifestyle because of the numerous benefits it has. The list of celebrities includes Ben Affleck, Miranda Kerr, Liv Tyler, and Hugh Jackman. They appreciate the positive effects of intermittent fasting which is very easy to follow.

Most celebrities prefer the Fast Diet version. According to many of their peers, they have enjoyed fantastic success with it. There was a very informative documentary on TV about this kind of lifestyle. Instead of searching for an exotic or little-known diet miracle, the Fast Diet is known to work because it has been tried and tested and found to be effective.

When celebrities are convinced that intermittent fasting provides a healthy lifestyle that can help them to lose weight and keep it off, then they are likely to adapt it. Plenty of celebrities fast in secret and do not wish to come out publicly. Others, such as Jimmy Kimmel, have spoken out publicly about intermittent fasting. They love this lifestyle because it is 100% natural and represents the way humans have been eating for thousands of years.

Other fans of this lifestyle include the wine and food editor Fiona Beckett from the British magazine, the Guardian. Even Kate Middleton's Uncle is trying one of the different protocols of intermittent fasting. Like many other fans of this lifestyle, he is of the opinion that it is making a huge difference in people's lives.

The Diet of Foodies

Intermittent fasting is also sometimes referred to as the diet of foodies. A foodie is simply anyone with a keen interest and finer taste for food, and sometimes wine. Foodies have gone through many different types of diets, many of which have not resulted in desired results.

For a long time, athletes and workouts enthusiasts were made to believe that eating five to six small meals was the best eating model. Others were made to fast for 24 hours or longer, but results and outcomes were not convincing and maintaining such lifestyle diets proved difficult. Most of them are now speaking quite positively about intermittent fasting. For foodies, it provides the ultimate flexibility in food choice. This means you can actually choose to enjoy generous amounts of high-calorie foods such as fast food, chocolate, rice, and so on.

You will still have to watch your calorie intake. All the aspects of intermittent fasting sound really awesome, easy for anyone to do, and manageable in the long run. Hunger is almost non-existent so intermittent fasting goes a long way in guaranteeing you success whatever benefits you may be seeking. Most diets often fail because of long hours of fasting and irresistible hunger. Intermittent fasting takes care of all the challenges encountered with other diets.

Chapter 2: Types of Intermittent Fasting

It has long been known that calorie restriction increases the lifespan of mammals. Research has revealed that intermittent fasting can provide the same benefits that regular calorie restriction does. Some health practitioners refer to it as under-nutrition without malnutrition.

Calorie restriction is the only experimental approach that always improves the survival rates of animals with cancer and extends lifespan by over 30%. However, researchers have noted that intermittent fasting is slightly more effective in certain health matters.

Many health experts think that it is a great idea to "starve" yourself a little each day or maybe a few days each week. This is because there is plenty of evidence that this is beneficial to the body and overall health. In fact, there are numerous benefits of managed food deprivation. There are different types of intermittent fasting protocols. Here are some of the most popular ones.

Different Types of Intermittent Fasting

Intermittent Fasting can be accomplished in a number of ways. This is because the aim is to fast for a period of time before eventually feasting on purpose. All you need to do is to consume some calories during a specific time of the day then choose when not to eat. Since intermittent fasting has become so popular in recent years, several different protocols have come up.All of them can be effective; your choice will be up to personal preference. Here are some of the more popular ones.

The 16-8 Protocol

This is one of the most common intermittent fasting protocols available. It requires you to fast for 16 hours within a 24-hour period, or a single day, and then have your meals within an 8-hour window. As an example, you may have your first meal at noon on day one then have your last one at 8.00 pm the same night. After your meal, ensure that you do not eat anything else for the next 16 hours. This means fasting until 12.00 pm the following day. However, there is no fixed starting time, so you may start and end the protocol any time you want.

With the 16-8 protocol, you can fit in two, three, or even four meals. This particular method is also known as the Leangains protocol. It can be as simple as choosing not to have anything to eat after dinner then skipping breakfast altogether. If your last meal was dinner at 9.00 pm one night, you would not have anything else to eat until 1.00 pm the following day. Technically, you will have fasted for 16 hours straight.

Health experts recommend that ladies fast for 14 to 15 hours only because they are better with shorter fasts compared to men. But people who feel hungry in the morning and treasure breakfast can have several cups of coffee, water, or green tea and other beverages to reduce the possibility of hunger pangs.

Ensure that you consume mostly healthy foods even as you switch to intermittent fasting. Eating junk food and excessive calories will not work very well with this kind of lifestyle. The 16-8 protocol is essentially the most natural method of intermittent fasting. Many people prefer it because it is almost effortless. In summary, the 16-8 protocol is best when you restrict your eating to an 8-10 hour window and fit in 2 to 3 meals. Make sure that you eat low-carbohydrate meals with plenty of vegetables and grains.

The 24-Hour Protocol

It is a well-known fact that we eat mostly when we are stressed, or feel lonely, frustrated, excited, confused, or even when we are happy. This means that we humans tend to eat in response to our emotions which is not the best approach to health, diet, or food intake. With this approach, we tend to feed our emotional hunger rather than psychological hunger.

Fortunately, the 24-hour protocol helps you to identify the difference between the two. For instance, if you have your last meal of the day at 8.00 pm one evening, then you will not eat anything for the next 24 hours. You do not have to follow this protocol every single day of the week. Instead, you can practice it once or twice each week.

Some people are unable to fast for 24 hours straight. Fortunately, these programs are flexible and so fasting for 18 or 20 hours is also acceptable. The main aim here is to find what works best for you and then learn to live with it. As you fast, you are allowed to drink a cup of coffee, black or green tea, and any other non-calorific beverages. If you are following this protocol for weight loss purposes, then you should maintain your regular eating habits.

Perform the 24-Hour Fast Once Each Week

Nutrition experts recommend that you perform this fast once a week. Find the day of the week when you are most sedentary then plan to fast that entire day. For instance, if your fast day is Tuesday, then start fasting on Monday after dinner. Do not eat any food all day until dinner time Tuesday.

The main challenge about this protocol is that many people are unable to maintain a fast for an entire 24-hour period. If this is you, then you do not have to fast for an entire 24 hours in the beginning. You can start with 14-16 hours then increase the hours until you can fast for a full 24 hours.

Sometimes fasting can cause practitioners to get angry and hungry. Those with conditions such as diabetes may not be able to cope with the 24-hour protocol. In such instances, participants are encouraged by health experts to modify this protocol or to choose a different one. This way, they will still be able to enjoy the benefits of fasting.

The 5:2 A.K.A FAST DIET

The most popular intermittent fasting protocol is the 5:2 diet also known as the fast diet. This particular protocol involves normal eating for five days per week then restricting calorie intake for two days of the week. This protocol was made popular by a British doctor and journalist, Michael Mosley.

This protocol is focus more of an eating pattern It requires the practitioner to restrict their calorie intake to 500 on fasting days. First, identify two non-consecutive days of the week and mark them as fast days. For instance, Monday and Thursday are preferred by most people.

On regular days, you should eat normally and without bingeing. You should also avoid junk foods as these will erode the great benefits of the fast. Plenty of women find this protocol much easier to follow than traditional diets.

Alternate-Day Fasting

The alternate-day fasting is another protocol of intermittent fasting. On this diet, you fast every other day, and then you eat whatever you want on non-fasting days. A modified version of this protocol involves eating about 500 calories on fasting days.

Alternate-day fasting is considered a very effective method of losing weight and also helps with numerous other health benefits as well. Your eating is restricted only half the time, yet the benefits are immense. During fasting days, you are allowed to drink as many beverages as you wish as long as they are calorie-free. For instance, you can have water, unsweetened tea, green tea, and coffee.

On the modified alternative-day fast, you are allowed to consume 20 – 25% of your energy requirements which is about 500 calories. Studies also indicate that women prefer this protocol compared to old-fashioned diets because the fast is broken each day and they get to choose foods that they like. The benefits of this particular protocol are just as great as those of other intermittent fasting protocols. Therefore, one protocol over others is only a matter of preference.

Studies have shown that people who follow intermittent fasting protocols may lose up to 8% of their body weight within 4 to 12 weeks. It was also discovered that this lifestyle is particularly effective as a weight loss tool among ladies aged between 40 and 60 years. Intermittent fasting and daily calorie restrictions are effective at reducing dangerous belly fat. The results are far better when compared to traditional fasting methods.

Combining intermittent fasting with endurance exercises can result in twice as much weight loss when compared to fasting on its own and more than six times more weight loss when compared to endurance workouts alone. The types of foods that you eat really do not matter because of the effectiveness of these fasting protocols. You can expect to enjoy excellent health benefits and improved appearance if you follow these protocols. Other benefits will be discussed in greater detail in a different chapter.

Spontaneous and Convenient Meal Skipping

There are other flexible forms of intermittent fasting. One of these is spontaneous meal skipping. This is a protocol that allows you to skip meals but only when it is convenient. You do not have to follow any of the structured intermittent fasting plans to actually see some benefits.

This form of intermittent fasting allows you to skip a meal from time to time such as when you are too busy, away somewhere, or not feeling very hungry. Many people think that they have to eat every few hours or they will suffer starvation. This is not true because the human body is designed to handle a prolonged period of hunger, not just skipping a meal or two.

Let us assume it's a Tuesday morning and you are not feeling hungry. You skipped breakfast that morning and headed off to work, then have a healthy lunch later. If you are traveling to a new place and cannot find something nutritious to eat, then skip the meal and wait to have a proper meal later.

This is not a complex or stressful form of fasting but a convenient one that comes with health benefits just like all the others.

Chapter 3: Benefits of Intermittent Fasting

The practice of intermittent fasting can lead to several metabolic changes in the body. These changes often begin within three to five hours after a meal once the body gets into the post-absorptive and not during digestion. Eating frequent meals means the body is constantly involved in a digestive activity.

People fast for various reasons such as religious, health, or medical purposes. However, anytime you deprive the body of nutrition, you allow your systems and organs to rest. Your body benefits immensely when these organs and systems take a break. These benefits are discussed in greater detail below.

What Happens to Your Body When You Fast

If you are planning to fast, then you need to understand what happens to your body during fasting. By understanding how fasting affects your body, you will be able to prepare yourself physically and mentally for it.

At the onset of fasting, you are likely to feel hungry. This is to be expected. Later in the day, you will experience a reduction in energy levels which might cause you to become moody and irritable. Those who prepare themselves mentally for the rigors of fasting cope much better than those who do not.

At a cellular level, your body is used to breaking down glucose from the food you eat to produce the energy that it needs to function properly. However, when you are fasting, your body still needs the energy to function normally. As such, your liver begins to convert fats and amino acids into glucose. Then your body will go into energy saving mode. Your blood pressure and heart rate will slow down, and you may feel drained. However, this will only last for about 10 to 15 minutes then your energy levels will return.

During fasting, your body will also go through a stage known as ketosis. This is the stage where the body starts to burn up fats stored in the body. Ketosis takes place, and you will then possibly stop feeling hungry. Ketosis is excellent for balancing blood sugar, weight loss, and much more.

Evidence-Based Benefits of Intermittent Fasting

1. Intermittent fasting helps you lose weight and belly fat for good!

When you fast, your body is not starved of glucose or energy needed to function. Instead, it taps into fat reserves that have accumulated in your body. These fats are accumulated by the body to be used where there is a scarce supply of food. Therefore, when you begin to fast, your body begins a slow but steady weight loss process which is hugely beneficial to your health.

Intermittent fasting is much more sustainable in the long run and more effective as a weight loss tool compared to crash diets. Numerous studies support intermittent fasting as a reliable option for weight maintenance and weight loss. You will notice considerable weight loss as you begin this lifestyle. Many people who try intermittent fasting also begin to consume fewer calories than before, even on days when they are not fasting.

Intermittent fasting enhances hormonal functions that support weight loss. The hormones that are released when you fast support the breakdown of body fat into glucose which is then used by the body as energy.

Essentially, intermittent fasting works on both ends of the calorie equation. It reduces the amount of food you consume while increasing your metabolic rate. When your metabolic rate goes up, your body becomes more efficient and stores less fat. You can expect to lose between 3% and 8% of your total body weight in 4 to 12 weeks. This is a significant amount of weight to lose in that period of time.

Although calorie counting is not necessary, weight loss when doing intermittent fasting is more as a result of reduced calorie intake. Therefore, intermittent fasting is an excellent lifestyle that can be adapted to help you restrict calories intake without necessarily trying to eat less. Numerous studies show it helps you lose weight and belly fat.

2. It helps regulate the function of hormones, genes, and cells

Intermittent fasting has been shown to regulate hormones and provide better hormonal balance in the body. During fasting, your organs get to rest, especially your liver, a crucial organ for naturally balancing hormones.

Insulin

Insulin is a hormone released by the pancreas that regulates the amount of sugar in the blood. When you fast, your body starts converting stored fats into energy to fuel cell activity. As a result, the body ends up with reduced amounts of stored fat. This makes muscles and cells more responsive to insulin, so the insulin in your body gets absorbed more.

With better absorption of insulin, your body is better able to regulate blood glucose. This is absolutely important as it helps prevent diabetes and also regulates glucose levels for those who may have the condition. As a woman, if you are searching for a natural method of increasing insulin sensitivity, then intermittent fasting provides an excellent solution for you. Generally, insulin resistance occurs as a result of excessive glucose amounts in body tissues, especially those not built for storage. When you fast, all this stored glucose gets consumed as energy, and your body once again functions normally.

Human growth hormone

This hormone is responsible for causing cells to divide and multiply. It also stimulates the synthesis of collagen in the tendons and skeletal muscles. HGH boosts the immune system and improves your physical capacity while breaking down lipids within the body to reduce body fat content. When you fast, you boost the levels of human growth hormone in your body up to 5 times. HGH has numerous benefits to your body which include weight loss, development of lean muscle, strong bones, healthy growth of hair, and many others.

Cortisol

This hormone is also known as the stress hormone. It is released into the body during emergency situations and triggers a flight or fight response together with the sympathetic nervous system. Intermittent fasting helps with the regulation of this stress hormone because it regulates insulin which is a cortisol antigen. When insulin is properly regulated, then there is very little cortisol in the body.

Female Hormones Estrogen

When there are high levels of estrogen in the body, issues such as headaches, irritability, and weight gain arise. There is an enzyme found in most tissues known as aromatase. This hormone converts testosterone into estrogen. Aromatase occurs in body fat, so people with high body fat often have elevated levels of estrogen. Reduced fat levels in the body result in lower aromatase levels in the body. This ensures less testosterone is converted to estrogen. Intermittent fasting, therefore, ensures adequate regulation of estrogen in the body. Prolonged fasting is not advisable, especially for women as it will negatively affect hormonal balance in the body.

Cells

Cells within your body often store fats and sometimes even disease-causing pathogens. When you fast, your body starts utilizing the fats stored in such cells. The process will also involve the elimination of other unwanted matter within the cells, including waste material and pathogens. When this happens, your cells undergo repair. This healing produces new cells that are more efficient, healthier, fat-free, and hence effective in carrying out normal but important functions.

3. Intermittent Fasting Reduces Risks of Type II Diabetes

One of the most serious conditions that many women suffer from is type II diabetes. The condition has become prevalent in the last couple of decades. This condition often occurs as a result of excess blood sugar due to insulin resistance. The body produces insulin to regulate the amount of glucose in the blood. However, when the body cannot regulate blood sugar properly, it causes diabetes which is a chronic condition that has no known cure. Insulin resistance results due to the accumulation of glucose in body tissue not designed to store fat.

Intermittent fasting has been proven to help the body eliminate excessive fat in the body and reduces insulin resistance. This leads to a significant reduction in glucose levels within the body. Human studies on individuals practicing intermittent fasting have shown a reduction in blood sugar levels by between 3% and 6%. Intermittent fasting has been shown to reduce damage to the kidneys which is often a result of the complications of type II diabetes. It normalizes blood sugar levels in the body. Basically, the effects of fasting can actually make a big difference in the way your body processes glucose. If you are looking for a natural way to increase insulin sensitivity, then intermittent fasting provides the best solution.

4. Boosts Metabolism

Intermittent fasting provides relief to your digestive system. Fasting on a regular basis boosts your metabolism so that your body burns fat more efficiently. This results in significant weight loss. For best results, try and combine fasting with regular workouts.

One of the best ways to improve your metabolism is to efficiently eliminate toxins and waste that accumulate due to ordinary drinking and eating. Intermittent fasting results in the cleansing of internal organs to increase metabolism. It also regulates your digestion and promotes healthy bowel function and hence improves the metabolic action.

When your metabolism slows down, the aging process kicks in. An efficient metabolism can slow down the aging process. Intermittent fasting gives your digestive system a break from normal digestion which slows down the aging process. Also when you improve your eating habits so that you only eat the right foods and in the correct quantity, you energize your metabolism which ensures it is efficient and functions properly.

Many experts are of the opinion that intermittent fasting has a lot more benefits compared to long-term calorie restriction which negatively affects the body's metabolism.

5. Extended Lifespan and Intermittent Fasting

Scientists at the University of Chicago have released findings of a study about intermittent fasting and longevity. The research reveals that intermittent fasting can delay the development of disorders that lead to death. There is evidence that shows that people who fast on a regular basis enjoy a healthier and longer life compared to people

The efficiency of metabolism in cells reduces over time especially when you consume 3 meals every single day. This tends to hasten the aging process. When you fast, you give the cells a break, so they rejuvenate and detoxify. This slows down the aging process considerably. Also, the cells are put in a state of mild stress whenever you fast which triggers the body to repair body cells and tissue and maintain them in excellent condition. These anti-aging properties help to keep your organs functioning efficiently and effectively.

6. Boosts the Immune System

The immune system is an important system within your body. It helps protect you against diseases, infections, and against dangerous pathogens. Scientists at the University of Southern California have demonstrated that fasting has the capability of regenerating the immune system. It triggers the production of new white cells which fight off infections and keep you free from infections and diseases.

Intermittent fasting allows your body to get rid of damaged, worn out, inefficient, or old cells of your immune system and replace them with newer immune system cells. Many researchers are of the opinion that intermittent fasting could greatly assist the elderly and anyone else with low immunity and prone to infections.

7. Excellent for Your Brain

Scientists often say that what is good for the body is also good for the brain. When you fast for relatively short periods of time, your metabolism will greatly improve. This will help reduce inflammation, oxidative stress, and blood sugar levels in the body. According to a study released in 2015 by the Society for Neuroscientists, it was shown that intermittent fasting has enormous health benefits for the brain.

When you fast, your brain is stimulated in various ways. Brain stimulation enhances memory performance, aids in recovery after brain injury, and promotes the growth of neurons. It also lowers the risks of brain conditions such as Alzheimer's and Parkinson's diseases. Research scientists have shown that intermittent fasting also improves quality of life and cognitive function of patients suffering from these brain conditions.

8. Helps to Combat Oxidative Stress

Oxidative stress is stress that is caused by unstable molecules within the body known as free radicals. Free radicals are very dangerous to the body and can be harmful. They normally interact with other important molecules in the body, react and cause long-term damage to cells and to organs inside your body.

Free radicals are harmful to the body and cause damage to your organs, DNA, protein, and cell membranes. They also enhance the aging process and can play a role in the onset or development of cancer and other health conditions. Intermittent fasting is a great solution to the problems caused by free radicals. Several studies show the benefits of intermittent fasting in enhancing the body's resistance to oxidative stress. When you fast, you activate stress defenses. These defenses are activated even if the stressor is not present. For instance, fasting activates the protein that maintains your DNA in great condition. During fasting, when the body begins breaking down fats in your cells as a source of energy, it also gets rid of waste within the cells as well as the free radicals. The cells get cleaned out, and rejuvenation process begins. Fasting also helps battle inflammation which is another major cause of various kinds of diseases.

9. Beneficial to Your Heart

Heart disease is the world's number one killer with millions of Americans falling victim each year. There are a number of risk factors or health markers that are largely associated with heart disease. These risk factors include blood triglycerides, inflammatory markers, total and LDL cholesterol, blood pressure, and blood sugar levels.

Researchers believe that intermittent fasting, or restricted calorie intake for a couple of hours once or twice a week greatly improves the risk factors associated with heart health. Fasting generally helps eliminate bad cholesterol or LDL cholesterol. It also helps reduce body weight. These are all factors that are considered high-risk indicators. Reduced bodyweight helps reduce your blood pressure while a reduction in LDL cholesterol helps reduce the risk of heart disease to your heart.

It has been known as a fact, for many years, that anyone who follows a certain lifestyle such as a restricted calorie intake once or twice a week will have better heart health compared to those who do not. Generally, people who fast often watch what they eat when they are not fasting and this translates into good weight control. Your levels of bad cholesterol decrease as you fast which is a good indicator of a healthy heart. As a whole, intermittent fasting has many heart benefits and ensures you have a healthy heart as well as very low-risk factors.

Calorie Restriction Benefits your Health

There are plenty of studies that have confirmed the immense benefits of calorie restrictions to your health. The studies also indicate that eating less is absolutely essential if you want to live longer. Research done in mice shows that life-long calorie restriction significantly alters the overall structure of gut microbiota. This alteration occurs in a manner that promotes longevity. One reason why calorie restriction lengthens lifespan is that of the positive effect it has on gut microbiota.

Increased longevity due to calorie restriction can be associated with a reduction in disease states that would otherwise end your life. Calorie restriction is also associated with several health improvements that include reduced inflammation, lower visceral fat levels, improved insulin sensitivity, and lower blood pressure levels. Previous research clearly demonstrated that calorie restriction helps to increase the lifespan of animals by inhibiting the mTOR pathway and improving insulin sensitivity.

Intermittent fasting has many benefits that are similar to calorie restriction, even when you do not strictly restrict the amount of calories you consume each day. This fact was demonstrated in a review conducted by research scientists in 2013. The review discovered a wide range of therapeutic benefits brought on by intermittent fasting even when there was no significant reduction in the total number of calories consumed. Basically, if you choose any intermittent fasting protocol, you can consume the same amount of calories as before and still enjoy the benefits of calorie restrictions.

Intermittent Fasting helps with the following;

- It reduces blood pressure levels
- Limits inflammation
- Promotes reduction in cellular damage and oxidative stress
- Improves metabolic efficiency
- Significant reductions in body weight for obese persons
- Prevent type II diabetes or slow down its progression
- Causes stem cells to enter a state of self-renewal
- Improves pancreatic function
- Protects against cardiovascular disease
- Modulate levels of dangerous visceral fats

Tips and Strategies for Managing Intermittent Fasting

- Drink green tea during fasting. While not essential, it makes the experience easier. Green tea suppresses appetite and curbs hunger pangs.
- It is important to drink water when you fast as it will fill your stomach. This sends a message to the brain that you are full and you will feel less hungry.
- Be on the lookout for body cues. For instance, if you feel upset or stressed out during your fast, then try to relax.

Take some deep breaths and focus closely because this is exactly what hunger does to you.

- Stock your house with healthy food options. Healthy foods include lean protein, veggies, and grains. These provide an excellent insurance policy so that you do not binge when you resume normal eating.

Chapter 4: Getting Started in Intermittent Fasting

By now you already understand that intermittent fasting is not a diet but a pattern of eating. It involves scheduling your meals such that you get the most out of them. You also know that intermittent fasting does not necessarily change *what* you eat but *when* you eat. It is very important that you change your eating times to allow a period of deliberate fast in your life.

You should change when you eat because this is a great way to get lean without drastically cutting down your calorie intake or going on a crazy diet. In fact, most women who start intermittent fasting often keep their calorie intake the same. Some of them opt to eat bigger meals within a shorter period of time. This type of lifestyle is a great way of maintaining your muscle mass while losing weight.

A Typical Intermittent Fasting Procedure

Take the example of Tiffany, from Albany, who has been practicing intermittent fasting for the last one year. She skips breakfast each day and then eats two meals the rest of the day. The first meal is at 1 PM while the second one around 8.00 pm. She then fasts for a total of 16 hours before having her next meal. While she follows this routine each day, you do not have to. One or two days a week is advisable.

However, since she started intermittent fasting and made it a lifestyle, Tiffany has noticed increased muscle mass and decreased body fat. Other notable changes include reduced training and workout times and increase energy and explosiveness. Basically, due to an intermittent fasting lifestyle, Tiffany became leaner, stronger, and fitter than ever before even though she eats less and works out less.

Getting Started with Intermittent Fasting

Intermittent fasting requires that you adjust your eating habits. Food is not deprived in this case, but you have to choose when to have your meals. When you begin practicing this lifestyle, you will have to deny yourself from food for a certain period during the day.

Remember that intermittent fasting is more of a lifestyle, so you need to understand what you are getting into. In most cultures, food is a huge part of life and our lives sort of circle around it. Therefore, choose a protocol that will suit your life. Several simple steps will help you get started. These are discussed below.

Choose your Preferred Intermittent Fasting Protocol

There are a number of protocols so find one that fits your life. For instance, if you are a morning person and enjoy working out followed by a snack right away, then find a protocol that is compatible with this kind of lifestyle. Some people love working out in the evenings and others mid-morning.

With today's tight schedules, you may want to fast or skip eating one or two days a week and get it out of the way, then not have to worry about fasting on the other days. For instance, you can choose to fast on Mondays and Thursdays and then lead a normal lifestyle for the remaining days.

Therefore, you can choose the eat-stop-eat protocol. This basically means on days when you fast, you eat early in the morning, fast for 16 hours and then resume eating normally. Other formats allow you to eat a maximum of 500 calories on fast days. This is actually on fast days if you cannot manage to do without food at all.

When choosing your preferred fasting protocol, you should consider other factors, such as the reasons why you are fasting. Most people fast to lose weight. However, some do it for religious reasons and others for health, diagnostics, and other reasons. There are those who simply need a simplified lifestyle. Others consider issues such as building muscle, anti-aging, quality of life, and even longevity.

If you fast only one day a week, you may not necessarily lose a lot of weight at once, but this protocol will help with weight maintenance and many other health benefits like longevity and blood sugar regulation.

Adjust your Eating Habits

It is advisable to consider adjusting your eating habits. One of the major benefits of intermittent fasting is that it mostly dictates when to eat but not what foods to eat. If you choose to eat healthy natural foods and avoid junk foods, then you will lose weight especially due to reduced calorie intake. A healthy diet and regular workouts are essential for weight loss and a healthy body.

Unhealthy eating habits can affect your energy levels, mood, blood sugar, and hormones whether you are fasting or not. It would be easier to make eating healthy a priority too. Otherwise, you will have to limit your eating window. Again, your body will have to work overtime trying to eliminate the toxins and junk that you take in.

A huge benefit of intermittent fasting is that, over time, your desire and appetite for unhealthy foods will diminish. Intermittent fasting is an excellent tool to help you manage the ill effects of unhealthy foods. Even then, cleaning up your diet or working towards it at the onset of your lifestyle change is very important.

Do your Research Thoroughly

There are plenty of different protocols that you can choose from. Before you choose one or the other, do as much research about it as possible. Find out what the specific benefits you will gain from choosing one protocol over the others and any drawbacks it may have.

You also need to understand everything you can about what intermittent fasting does to your body, your mind, and your life. When you understand the kind of lifestyle you are getting into and the benefits you stand to gain, then you will be able to persevere and eventually practice intermittent fasting happily and diligently. Some of the protocols you may want to look at include;

- Eat-stop-eat protocol
- The 24-hour protocol
- The fast diet
- The 16-8 protocol
- The 5:2 fast diet
- The alternate-day fasting
- The every-other-day protocol

What you need to do is try out some of these intermittent fasting protocols and find the one that works best for you. Try and make it a lifestyle that you can practice for the long run. You can also alternate from one protocol to another periodically.

Begin the Transition

Now begin the transition into a lifestyle that includes fasting on a regular basis each week. What you should now do is ease into your chosen protocol. This means doing things such as delaying your first meal of the day and cutting back on late night eating.

Remember that intermittent fasting is a lot more about the mind as it is about diet and lifestyle. You need to train your mind to adjust to your chosen lifestyle. For instance, delaying breakfast by about an hour and stopping your evening meals an hour earlier helps train your mind about the impending lifestyle change. This is the same way that muscles are trained. You start with a lighter weight and gradually increase the weight as your strength increases.

Now your intermittent fasting journey has started. The process will involve on-going modifications regarding your eating habits, diet, and fasting times until you note the results that you want and are comfortable with the lifestyle changes. For obese and overweight women, it is a good idea to adjust your eating habits and restrict the eating window between six and eight hours. This way, the body gets plenty of opportunities to rest and lose weight at a rapid yet comfortable rate.

Find a Support Person or Group

One of the best ways of being successful with this lifestyle is to identify other persons, especially women, who are on the same journey. Social media websites such as Facebook are great places to find support groups. There are a number of pages specifically set up on Facebook for women who practice intermittent fasting.

Apart from social media networks, you can find platforms where people are leading a similar lifestyle frequent. For instance, forums like bodybuilding.com are full of men and women who have adopted intermittent fasting as a lifestyle. You can also share your lifestyle changes with people close to you such as your partner, kids, workmates, a neighbor, and anyone else you consider close. This is because intermittent fasting may be a little bit challenging, to begin with, and you will require the understanding and patience of those around you.

Consider Cutting Down Workouts and Adjusting the Hours

In the beginning, you may encounter numerous challenges while coping with hunger and working out. This is because your body is not yet used to this lifestyle. However, you should not give up. Instead, think about making appropriate adjustments. For instance, you may go for walks instead of jogging. This way, you will manage to handle the challenges experienced during the initial stages.

Rest assured that your energy levels will get back to normal once this transition period is over. You will then realize that you can work harder than you did before. In the beginning, though, your limbs will feel weak, and you might lack the motivation to workout. Your hunger pangs will also rise. Learn to persevere and be strict with your eating window. It will be a good idea if this eating window comes right after your workout sessions.

You can adjust your workouts so that you start earlier or later than usual. Many people prefer their workouts to be within their fasting window to distract from the hunger. Others need to get the workouts scheduled to time the end of the fasting window, so they do not suffer from hunger afterward. Your workouts should be timed to suit your preferences, schedule, and priorities.

Consider the Use of Delayed Gratification

Delayed gratification is a simple process that works great when you start fasting. Consider a little child who asks its mom permission to go to the playground to play with other kids. Instead of a direct yes, the mother is likely to delay the approval to a later moment. The delay eases the pain of desire. You can consider delayed gratification as an excellent tool to help you handle your intermittent fasting lifestyle especially when you start feeling hungry.

In the course of each day, you are likely to be offered a snack by co-workers or see the delicious cereal and milk your child, or family member is eating. Your mouth may water and your heart filled with the desire to eat. Using the delayed gratification tactic, you can promise yourself the treat, not at that moment though but at a later time. You can consider putting this down on a piece of paper or diary to remind yourself how strong you are and how far you have come.

Re-organize your Meals

It is a good idea to consider rearranging your meals just so that you eat your complex carbs and protein first. Your list needs to contain foods such as vegetables, fruits, lean meat, fish, grains, and other healthy options. Choose foods that are high in nutrients to nourish your body adequately.

Try and organize your meals ahead of time. When you prepare your meals, remember to include a complex carbohydrate and protein. It is possible that by the time you get to your eating window, you will be hungry enough, so a ready meal after working out is always welcome. The order of your meals should first be proteins, followed by complex carbs, then simple carbs, and finally any delayed gratification foods.

Exercise while Fasting

You can also try out exercising during the fasting window. Working out during your fasting period is common with most women as they can burn more calories this way. Exercising during your fasting window is sometimes referred to as fasted training. You can try it and see if it works out for you. If not, then you can workout during your eating window.

When you workout during your fasting window, your insulin levels will be low. This means your body will not derive energy from the food that you eat but from stored fat. There are plenty of women who prefer working out on empty due to inherent benefits like the ability to burn more body fat. This helps to get rid of stubborn fat stored in the body.

Take a Before Photo

One other thing you may want to consider is taking a before photo. While it is not an essential aspect of intermittent fasting, it can provide a great reference point especially if one of your goals is to lose weight. Having these photos taken will help keep you motivated. You can continue taking photos after a couple of weeks into the fast to observe and note any significant changes.

Taking a before and after photo will help you monitor progress, especially if you are trying to lose belly fat or build muscle. As you fast, and workout, your body releases more HGH or human growth hormone. This hormone will help your body to develop lean, toned muscles over time. A progress photo will serve as an excellent motivation tool that will help you to keep focused on your weight loss goals.

The Bottom Line

What you need to keep in mind is that intermittent fasting is one of the most effective and successful lifestyle changes you will ever make in your life. However, getting started is the most challenging part. As a matter of fact, the first 10 days to 2 weeks will probably be the toughest yet. The good thing is that once you get used the lifestyle, you will easily get used to it and begin to enjoy the benefits shortly thereafter. You will be shocked at the drastic decrease in the cravings that you currently have, especially for junk foods and fast food.

Chapter 5: Intermittent Fasting Differences Between Men and Women

Nutritional Considerations for Women

By now you probably understand what intermittent fasting is all about and its benefits for weight loss and your overall health. For women, there are a few things that you need to know because fasting can affect you in ways that are different from men.

Many women who have tried intermittent fasting acknowledge its numerous benefits. These include reduced risks of heart disease, gaining lean muscle, recommended blood sugar levels, reduced risk of chronic diseases such as cancer and many others.

However, women need to be aware of hormonal changes within their bodies and how these changes are affected by fasting and an active lifestyle. The major concern often has to with women's fertility hormones and fasting. Fortunately, this concern has been adequately addressed, and women can safely fast.

Women and Nutrition Deficiency

In women, calorie restriction due to lifestyle changes like fasting can alert the body to interrupt fertility. Anytime you suffer a low-calorie or low-fat diet, your body adopts a defensive mechanism which is only discarded when sufficient nutrition intake resumes. While fasting can affect your hormones, intermittent fasting does support proper hormonal balance leading to a healthy body and weight loss the right way.

Why Do Women Fast?

There are many reasons why women fast. Most of these reasons relate to weight loss, better health, improved physical appearance, and fat loss in certain areas such as the tummy and waist. Some women chose to fast to lead a healthy lifestyle and others to manage different medical conditions like high blood pressure, diabetes, and even cancer.

Fasting Challenges that Women Experience

Some women who fast regularly experience a number of challenges. For instance, some women claim to experience problems such as metabolic disturbances, early-onset menopause, and missed periods.

When a woman's body suffers hormonal issues and fertility problems, this could lead to hair loss, pale skin, a lack of energy, acne, and similar challenges. Fortunately, you do not have to suffer any such challenges as a woman. You can tailor your eating and fasting periods so that they match your lifestyle and enable you to avoid the issues and challenges that affecting fasting women.

Fasting and Your Hormones

When done incorrectly, intermittent fasting can result in hormonal imbalances in women. This is because women are extremely sensitive to what scientists refer to as signals of starvation. When the body senses that it is being starved of important nutrients, it produces excessive amounts of the hunger hormones ghrelin and leptin. It is the production of these hormones that causes fasting women to experience insatiable hunger.

Why Does Fasting Affect Women's Hormones?

Scientists are not a 100% sure why women's hormones are affected so much compared to men's. However, suspicion points to a protein known as kisspeptin. This molecule is used by neurons for communicating with each other. It is also super-sensitive to insulin, leptin, and ghrelin, which are all hormones that control hunger.

It is interesting to note that women have more kisspeptin neurons than men. More of this molecule means greater sensitivity to alterations in energy balance. This is probably the reason why fasting causes the production of this molecule to dip, hunger hormones are not as properly regulated.

Do Not Ignore Hunger Cues

When the body produces excessive hormones that prompt you to eat, you are likely to ignore them. Apparently, many women ignore these hunger signals, so the signals get even more intense. The problem is that even these loud signals are ignored, and this might lead to bingeing later on, followed by another under-eating and starvation period. This vicious cycle will continue and is likely to throw your hormones out of whack and possibly even affect your overall health altogether.

Fasting and Hormones in Women

Metabolism and female health are strongly interconnected. If, as a woman, you are experiencing physical and physiological challenges, then your health could be affected. Fortunately, regular fasting, working out, and eating a healthy diet can help resolve the health challenges. Intermittent fasting has been shown to help balance hormones in women's bodies and ensuring proper functioning of organs and systems in your body.

Women tend to consume less protein compared to men. It follows then that fasting women consume even less protein. Less consumption of protein results in fewer amino acids in the body. Amino acids are essential for the synthesis of insulin-like growth factor in the liver which activates estrogen receptors. The growth factor IGF-1 causes the uterine wall lining to thicken as well as the progression of the reproductive cycle.

Take Enough Protein

You need to note that low protein intake can affect some of your hormones such as estrogen. There are estrogen receptors located throughout your body including bones, intestinal tract, and the brain. The metabolic function in your body will change if the estrogen balance is affected. This will affect your digestion, mood, bone formation, cognition, and so much more.

Even in the brain, estrogen stimulates neurons that stop the production of appetite-regulating chemicals. Basically, if you do anything to cause estrogen drop in your body, then you could end up feeling seriously hungry and eating a lot more than you would normally. This, therefore, means that estrogens are the key regulators of metabolism. These are probably the reasons why women, in general, tend to find it harder to lose weight and shed off pounds.

The Best Intermittent Fasting Approach for Women

Women are more sensitive to hunger signals than men. When these signals are released by the body, fasting can become a challenge. Fortunately, this can be addressed by consuming less than 500 calories of healthy, nutritious foods. This small meal will keep hunger pangs at bay and will enable your body to regulate hormones while keeping calorie intake at a minimum.

Try Crescendo Fasting

One of the solutions put forward by doctors is a fasting protocol known as crescendo fasting. This protocol has been designed specifically for women. For women, you should not fast every single day of the week but rather, only one or two days each week.

Women benefit a lot more when they only fast once or twice a week rather than every single day. This enables you, as a woman, to benefit from intermittent fasting but without any hormonal imbalance. This kind of approach is a lot gentler on your body and will ensure you easily adapt to regular fasting.

Benefits of Crescendo Fasting

There are numerous benefits of this fasting protocol. However, the most important of these include;

- You gain energy
- Improving inflammatory markers
- Losing weight and body fat
- No hormonal challenges

Rules for Crescendo Fasting

1. Fast only 2 or 3 days a week on non-consecutive days. For instance, fast on Tuesdays, Fridays, and Sundays.
2. Fast for 12 to 16 hours only. Do not exceed 16 hours if you can help it.
3. On your fasting days try and do some workouts such as yoga or walking.
4. On other days, do heavier workouts such as cardio or weight training.
5. You are allowed to take lots of water, tea, and coffee as long as they are free of added sugar, sweeteners, or milk.
6. Consider taking 5 – 8 grams of BCAA (branch chain amino acids) on your fast days. They contain very little calories yet provide much-needed fuel to your muscles. These amino acids also take the edge off hunger and fatigue.

Additional Tips

You may want to consider having a cup of coffee instead of an 18-hour dry fast. You can add some grass-fed butter and coconut oil. Have this for breakfast but without any protein or carbohydrates. If you feel hungry later on in the day, you can brew another cup.

The fat-burning process keeps your body in a state of ketosis so that you enjoy all the cell renewing benefits associated with intermittent fasting. Your brain receives sufficient energy so that you do not suffer from stress. With this approach, you enjoy the same energy levels from a normal breakfast but without having to consume any food. You will not even have to think about food until later on in the day.

This approach to fasting tells your body that it is time for the cells to burn fat to obtain energy and to clean house. Crescendo fasting is a game changer for women. It will additionally boost your fertility and attractiveness. Within a couple of weeks, you will note the following benefits;

- Radiant skin
- Healthy libido
- Shiny hair
- An energetic demeanor
- Appropriate body weight

If you are aged 40 and above or happen to be overweight, then you may want to add grass-fed collagen to your morning cup of coffee on fasting days. Collagen may spike your hunger a little but will definitely reset your leptin which is one of the hunger hormones.

Keep your sugars and fructose levels to a minimum to optimize leptin levels in the body. If you do not like coffee, you can drink warm water or another beverage to keep your mind off hunger.

Nutritional Concerns for Men

While there are numerous concerns for women who are considering intermittent fasting, men who consider the practice typically have far less to worry about. In fact, generally speaking, the only men who need to be hesitant about starting an intermittent fasting diet are those who are already underweight or are currently dealing with, or have previously dealt, with eating disorder issues. Men who are diabetic or hyperglycemic should also avoid intermittent fasting unless their insulin or blood sugar levels are well-regulated. Even then, it is crucial that you monitor your levels closely and stop fasting as soon as an issue arises.

Generally speaking, intermittent fasting is known to have a generally beneficial impact on lipids in the body, noticeably reducing glucose, triglyceride levels and cholesterol levels in men. Additional health benefits in men are known to include increased lifespan, increased testosterone, decreased bad cholesterol, improved weight loss reduced blood pressure, reduced effects of aging, decreased inflammation, increased amounts of human growth hormone (HGH) and reduced risk of chronic disease.

Intermittent fasting and testosterone

Men who are looking to pack on the muscle mass have another reason to strongly consider some variation of intermittent fasting and that is because of the benefits it causes when it comes to natural testosterone production. It is a well-documented fact that testosterone plays a noticeable role in the development of muscle size and mass. What is less common knowledge, however, is the fact that eating anything more than 300 calories in a single go will actually decrease the amount of testosterone that their bodies produce for three hours or more.

While this is not to say that not eating boosts testosterone levels, it is accurate to say that by not eating for a prolonged period of time, men who are looking to maximize their daily intake of testosterone will see better results when they fast for prolonged periods of time as, after 300 calories, the additional decrease in testosterone causes negligible additional losses.

What's more, a 1989 study found that men who fasted prior to exercising saw nearly a 200 percent increase in their body's natural ability to utilize the testosterone they already had access to. Another study from around the same time found that after 24 hours of consuming no calories, growth hormone levels were elevated 2000% from the baseline. Growth hormone rises in correlation with testosterone and is highly anabolic.

Essentially what these studies mean is that intermittent fasting increases testosterone while at the same time stimulating the correct group of hormones to support additional healthy testosterone production as well. As such, men who are interested in maximizing their hormonal health may find that intermittent fasting is an ideal way to go about doing so.

Losing Man Boobs with Intermittent Fasting

Another great thing about intermittent fasting is that it can help men remove the, if not disturbing, annoying man boobs. Intermittent fasting, for emphasis, has been proven to be effective in reducing body fat – more effective than low calorie diets.

Intermittent fasting can reduce the fat in the body in multiple mechanisms:

Growth Hormone Increased

The most powerful hormones in our body that burn fats are growth hormone. In a study, 24-hour fast has been proven to increase the growth hormone in men by 2000%.

Insulin Sensitivity Increased; Insulin Levels Decreased

The most essential regulator of fat metabolism is insulin. When you have high levels of insulin, your body finds it difficult to break down fats. A study has found that intermittent fasting can reduce 57% of insulin levels.

This means intermittent fasting reinforces the body to become a better fat-burning machine. Hence, fats from the foods you eat are less likely to be stored in the body.

Inflammation is reduced

Men with higher levels of estrogen – technically, those with man books, have high levels of chronic inflammation in the body. High chronic inflammation in the body could mean to more difficulty in getting rid of man books and losing weight.

Studies found that intermittent fasting reduces chronic inflammation in the body. Hence, men who fast are more likely to be able to get rid of man boobs.

65

Intermittent fasting indeed is a great diet program not only for women but also for men. It offers a plethora of health benefits that not only will make you leaner, but also physically and mentally healthy.

Chapter 6: Nutrition During Intermittent Fasting

Another crucial point you need to keep in mind is that good nutrition is essential. Eating a balanced diet is vital for good health and well being. Proper nutrition provides your body with all the vitamins, protein, energy, minerals, and essential fats it requires.

Nutrition and Food

Nutrition is the science of nutrients found in food and the relationship between nutrients and good health, reproduction, growth, and disease. According to the US government national library of medicine, nutrition is about eating a healthy and balanced diet. It is almost impossible to talk about healthy nutrition without talking about different kinds of food and planning your meals.

A healthy diet refers to nutrition, food preparation, and storage methods that preserve the nutrients appropriately. An unhealthy diet can result in diseases such as scurvy, anemia, even blindness. It can also result in chronic conditions such as high blood pressure, heart conditions, and diabetes.

Even as you practice intermittent fasting, you need to ensure that your diet consists of a wide variety of different foods. This way, your body will receive the essential nutrients it requires for growth and good health. However, your food intake will depend on a couple of factors such as your reasons for fasting.

Remember that the intermittent fasting lifestyle does not really limit what you eat but guides your diet to ensure you get the benefits of a healthy diet.
If you regularly consume a healthy diet even as you fast, then you will experience some or all of the following benefits

- Stubborn fat loss
- Weight loss
- Lower blood pressure
- Reduced risk of chronic illnesses

Always remember to keep food quality as high as possible. Eat only nutritious meals that will nourish your body. Watch the calories and keep them low. Never try to compensate for the calories you missed during fasting. Also, stay committed to the cause and stick with it for an extended period of time.

Regular Meals and Nutrition

The nutrition that you need is derived from the meals that you consume so it is important to first plan your meals then focus on the content of the meals. Ignoring meal planning means you are likely to lose out on some of the essential benefits of an intermittent fasting lifestyle.

High-protein Foods

Some of the foods that are high in energy and protein include the following;

- eggs
- meat
- nuts
- Fish that are high in omega-3s such as mackerel and salmon
  full-fat dairy products like cheese and yogurt

Now, this lifestyle demands that you fast regularly then have your meals within the limited eating window. For example, if you are basing your fasting on the 16-8 protocol, you will fast for a total of 16 hours and restrict your meals to the 8-hour eating window.

When it comes to determining how you are going to break down your meals for the day, it is important to keep in mind that intermittent fasting does not worry about how you break up your calories during your non-fasting hours, as long as you keep them to the predetermined window and do not overdo it in the process. With that being said, you may find it easier mentally, to stick to less than three meals during your non-fasting periods to ensure that you do not accidentally undo all of your hard work in the process.

Eat breakfast or dinner, but not both

Skipping breakfast a couple of times a week is an excellent idea to incorporate into your lifestyle. There are those who are inclined to have breakfast each day and simply cannot handle a morning without their favorite cereal. If that describes you, then feel free to have breakfast and lunch, then skip dinner.

Remember, it does not matter what time your non-fasting period starts and ends, as long as you stick to the same cycle every day to ensure that your body has the time it needs to get used to this new way of eating. If you spend too much time mixing things up, you will likely find that your body shuts down its weight loss completely while it tries to figure out just what exactly is going on. If you want to change to a different type of intermittent fasting, give your body a week or two of normal eating first.

Always fill up your plate with low-calorie vegetables

These types of vegetables taste great, fill your stomach, and do your body a lot of good.

Opt for higher protein meals. Higher protein meals help you to feel full for much longer periods of time. Protein is also high in calories so do not have too much of it. However, you can make it your main source of calories.

Keep your carbohydrates to a minimum

This is because carbohydrates are quite high in calories and will make you feel hungry again pretty soon. Carbohydrates include breakfast cereals, sweet potatoes, pasta, rice, potatoes, sweet corn, and bananas among many others.

Do not be afraid of Fat

While fat may be high in calories, it helps to make you feel full. You should include small amounts of fat in all your meals, especially on fast days. While the recommended amount for women is 500 calories, it is not wrong if you take a little extra. You can also consider taking ready-made meals. All you need to do is to ensure these meals are low in sugar and carbohydrates yet high in vegetables and proteins.

Dietary Concerns

You should keep your meals modest in size yet rich in nutrients. If you consume a large meal after the fast, your body will focus on digesting the meal and shut off fat burning. A large meal is also not ideal for mid-morning or the afternoon. It will probably make you lethargic and tired. Large meals in the course of the day are not effective at limiting hunger. You can break your fast with a small meal of about 400 to 500 calories. The meal should include fruit, protein, and some healthy fats.

Keep careful watch on your protein

Standard wisdom means says that you are going to want to take in between 20 and 30 grams of protein every four hours while you are awake. While intermittent fasting makes this unattainable, you are still going to want to take in between 80 and 120 grams of protein per day. If you are planning a serious strength workout then you are going to want to do so between two snacks, if not two full meals.

It is also important to keep in mind that a snack or two, now and then, can be extremely beneficial either before or after you exercise, assuming your variation of intermittent fasting supports them, of course. A snack or a meal that is consumed around three hours before you exercise, assuming it is high in protein, should provide you with the fuel you need to make it through an average workout. You will want to shorten this window to no more than two hours if you discover that you are prone to low blood sugar.

These meals should include blood-sugar stabilizing protein along with fast-acting carbs, for example two pieces of toast with banana slices and peanut butter. Additionally, sometime in the two hours after your workout you are going to want to try and consume approximately 20 grams of protein and 20 grams of carbs to ensure maximum muscle growth and to get your glycogen stores up high enough that you maintain energy until it is time to eat again.

Count the amount of calories that you need

Ideally you will want to be sure to consume a majority of your daily caloric intake in the period immediately following your workout period. This will not only make it easier for your body to generate lean muscle mass it will also make it easier to recover from the workout. In order to do this, you are going to want to start by determining the caloric requirements your body needs in order to build muscle.

To do so, you are going to need to determine your basal metabolic rate (BMR) which is the number of calories you burn while resting. The more lean muscle mass you have, the higher your BMR is going to be. Essentially what this means is that the more muscular physique you have, the more calories you are going to be burning around the clock. The average human body burns about 60 percent of its daily calorie consumption just through natural daily processes. From there, the body burns about 30 percent of its energy on physical activity and 10 percent on digestion.

To determine how many calories your body burns while resting, you can use the following formula. First you will need to determine your weight in kilograms by dividing your current weight by 2.2. You will also need to determine your height in centimeters which can be found by taking your height in inches and multiplying by 2.54.

For men, your BMR will be equal to 66.47+(13.75 x weight in kilograms) + (5 x height in centimeters) – (6.75 x age).

For women, your BMR is going to be equal to (65.09 + (9.56 x weight in kilograms) + (1.84 x height in centimeters) – (4.67 x Age).

The end result is the number of calories you burn while your body is at rest. For example, for a man who weighs 200 lbs. their BMR would be about 2,200 calories. From there, you are going to want to use the Sterling-Pasmore Equation to determine how many calories you need based on your current amount of lean body mass. Each pound of lean muscle mass requires 13.8 calories to support it. You can determine your current lean body mass from standard body fat measurements.

Calculate lean muscle mass vs. fat mass:
Body fat % x scale weight= fat mass
Scale weight - fat mass= lean body mass

Once you have determined your BMR, you will want to account for the additional calories that are burned through exercise.

- If you live a primarily sedimentary lifestyle you will want to multiply your BMR by 1.2.

- If you perform a light exercise routine 3 or 4 times per week you you will want to multiply your BMR by 1.375.

- If you perform moderate exercise between 3 and 5 days per week you will want to multiply your BMR by 1.55.

- If you exercise at a moderate intensity 6 or 7 days a week you will want to multiply your BMR by 1.725.

- If you are extremely active and exercise 6 or 7 days a week for 90 minutes or more you will want to multiply your BMR by 1.9.

With your BMR in mind, you are then going to want to consume about 20 percent of those calories before you exercise for the best results. This meal or snack should be a quality mix of both carbs and protein. Then, when you are finished exercising you are going to want to consume about 60 percent of your total calories sometime in the next 2 to 4 hours. This might seem like a lot but if you focus on calorie dense foods it should not be a problem.

Additionally, with this type of setup it is important to keep in mind that you are typically better off focusing on a diet with more carbs and less fat to support muscle growth. This is due to the fact that, following a workout, you are going to want to focus on carbs instead of fats which can be detrimental. This does not mean you are going to want to eliminate all fats, it just means you are going to want to limit the number of fats you consume in your post-workout meals.

If you lead a mostly sedimentary lifestyle then you will want to take in about 31 calories per kilogram per day to maintain your weight. If you are a recreational athlete then this number will be between 33 and 38 calories. If you are an endurance athlete then this number will be between 35 and 50 calories based on your training. If you are strength training and exercising heavily then this will be between 30 and 60 calories based on your training.

If you are looking to build muscle mass then you are going to want to ensure that you take in an additional 250 to 500 calories per day depending on the type of exercise you are doing. On the other hand, if you are exercising on a daily basis and are looking to lose weight then you should subtract an additional 300 calories from your daily intake. This will help you to not only lose weight, but also to maintain muscle mass in the process.

Number of meals during Intermittent Fasting

What is the ideal number of meals to take on fasting days? How about other days? There are numerous answers to these questions, but to optimize your lifespan and reduce your risk of getting any chronic diseases, you should personally choose the fasting and eating plan that best suits your circumstances.

For a long time, we believed in the adage of eating three square meals per day, every day, with snacks in between, to maintain optimum insulin and blood sugar levels. However, mounting evidence continues to show that this continuous eating is contributing to the problem of obesity and endemic conditions such as diabetes.

Continuous eating also wears down the digestive system and internal organs. This tends to speed up the aging process. By giving your digestive system and internal organs a chance to rest, you add years to your life and slow down the aging process. The biggest risk of spreading your meals from morning to noon and evening is overeating. Other not-so-obvious problems include some biological changes that occur and cause metabolic dysfunction, poor health, and weight gain.

From a historic perspective, we know that our ancestors did not have access to food 24-hours a day every single day. They probably ate once or twice a day and then went for long periods without any food. As a matter of fact, there is evidence about numerous benefits that take place in your cells, organs, and systems when you go for long stretches without food.

Applying Nutrition Knowledge to your Diet

Eat breakfast or dinner, but not both:

Skipping breakfast a couple of times a week is a great idea to incorporate into your lifestyle. However, there are some who feel compelled to have breakfast each morning. If that is you, then you can have breakfast and lunch, then skip dinner.

Those with physically tasking jobs are better off having a solid breakfast and lunch, then doing without dinner. The important point to remember here is to try and have your meals within a six to eight-hour window and to avoid any meals or snacks just before retiring to bed at night. As long as you have your meals within the eight-hour window, then you can choose between which two meals to have. You can have breakfast and lunch or lunch and supper. Try as much as possible, to avoid having both breakfast and dinner.

It is important to observe the three-hours-before-bed rule. For instance, if you go to bed at 11.00 pm, then you should have your last meal of the day by 8.00 pm. Please note that all these diet and meal plans are suitable only for adult women. Young people need to eat three square meals a day and snacks in between as they expend a lot of energy every day and their bodies are still developing.

Also, all meals in your diet and meal plans should revolve around real food. This means fresh fruits and vegetables, whole grains, lean meats, salads, white meat, legumes, and all other natural foods. Avoid junk food, sugary beverages, fizzy drinks, and unhealthy snacks. Instead, drink plenty of water, fruit and vegetable juices, and soups.

Nutrition Tips for a Healthy Body

It is advisable to ensure you have at least three hours after your last meal of the day before finally retiring to bed. There are good reasons for this. The three-hour window ensures no digestion takes place as you sleep. This will help prevent cell damage and optimize your mitochondrial functions. It also ensures that you avoid chronic degenerative diseases like diabetes, cancer, heart disease, and high blood pressure among others. You will instead live a long and healthy, disease-free life.

1) **Energy production in the body**

To understand the reasons why you need to avoid late night meals, you should first learn how your body produces energy. Your cells contain organelles known as mitochondria which are responsible for producing energy from the food that you consume. Mitochondria live within the cells of your body and are optimized to generate energy that your body requires to function.

Each cell contains between 100 and 100,000 mitochondria. The mitochondria work effectively to produce energy. They produce energy by generating and transferring electrons to ATP within your body. When you have excessive amounts of food in your system or are insulin resistant, then your body will become dysfunctional.

This is likely to cause dysfunctional cells which then contribute to DNA mutations in your body, causing lasting damage to your cell membranes. A lot of scientists and health experts believe that the damage caused by these electrons is one of the major reasons for premature aging. To avoid these complications within your body, you should resolve any insulin resistance challenges you may have.

Also, ensure that you finish all your meals early enough and not eat at night. When you sleep that your body needs the least amount of calories. If you feed mitochondria when you sleep, then your body will generate excessive free radicals that will contribute to chronic diseases, damage your tissue, and accelerate aging.

Intermittent fasting provides one of the best remedies for people suffering from insulin resistance. It provides a powerful intervention and will help restore your health within a relatively brief period of time. This is also another great reason why it is sometimes advisable to skip dinner rather than breakfast.

2) Drink water before meals

According to reports based on the latest research, drinking about 500 ml of water, or about 2 glasses of water, can help you lose weight. In the study, obese participants who drank at least 500 ml before each meal lost at least 3 pounds more than other participants in the course of three months. All participants in the study received weight management consultation with health experts on how to exercise and improve their diets.

On average, participants lost almost 9.5 pounds or 4.3 kilos during the 3-month duration of the study. This study makes sense as thirst is sometimes confused with hunger. Also, after drinking water, you are bound to feel full, so you are likely to eat less. Those who drank 500ml of water only once a day lost on 1.75 pounds or 0.8 kilos in the same period.

3) Should You Drink Coffee When Fasting

It is okay to drink coffee when you are fasting. Having two or three cups of coffee while fasting will reduce your appetite, make you feel good, and accelerate your metabolism. Should you be working out later in the day, then the coffee will positively affect your stamina and strength.

The effects of a cup of coffee last for about 6 hours. This means that even if you intend to workout later in the day, you should still get an extra kick from the morning cup of coffee. Also, coffee has numerous health benefits and is a rich source of antioxidants.

Chapter 7: Exercise and Intermittent Fasting

The benefits of intermittent fasting can be enhanced through exercise and regular workouts. Therefore, if you are practicing intermittent fasting, then you should adapt a regular workout regime. But what do exercises look like when you are fasting? This depends on a couple of factors. For instance, what exercises do you do on fasting days and non-fasting days? Which intermittent fasting protocol are you following? Also important is how your body responds to workouts during fasting sessions.

Adding exercise to an intermittent fasting plan

Food is the fuel that your body uses to power itself and to build new muscle when exercising. With that in mind, it shouldn't be surprising that when you eat or do not eat can easily have a serious impact both on how easily you will find a given workout and also how effective that workout will be.

It does not matter if you are training for endurance or training to improve your strength, your body primarily uses the glycogen found in stored carbohydrates to fuel your exercise. However, when your glycogen reserves are running low, such as when you are in the latter half of a period of fasting, then your body is going to need to look to other energy sources like fat to power your exercise routine. This means that you are likely to burn up to 20 percent more fat if you exercise during a fast as opposed to just after you have broken one.

Unfortunately, this isn't purely good news as if glycogen is in short supply your body is more likely to burn protein, in addition to fat, in order to keep your bodily processes working as they should. As protein is also responsible for building healthy muscles, if you do not take the proper precautions you can find yourself losing muscle mass as well as fat, if you exercise while fasting.

This won't just affect how much you can bench press or how toned your body looks, it will also slow your metabolism which will make it more difficult for you to lose weight in the long run as your body naturally adapts to the number of calories you are consuming on a regular basis over time. As such, once your body gets used to the fact that you are consuming fewer calories per day on average your body will eventually get used to burning fewer calories each day to ensure that you have enough energy left over for the basics such as staying healthy, breathing and even staying upright throughout the day. It will typically take about a month of regular rounds of fasting for your body to adapt to the change.

When it comes to merging your existing exercise plan with intermittent fasting, it is important to also keep in mind that all types of exercise are going to be more difficult than normal if you are exercising on an empty stomach as your blood sugar and glycogen levels will naturally be low which means that you are going to also feel weaker than normal as well. As such, it is important to schedule your works at the end of your fast, or during your meal times, to ensure you aren't depriving your body of the tools it needs to take advantage of your hard work.

Tips for exercising effectively

1) **Low intensity is key**

If you plan on exercising regularly while you are fasting, it is important to limit your cardio to low-intensity options. This means you should still be able to carry on a conversation with relative ease if you are exercising during a fast. This means you are going to want to stick to things like a light jog or 15 minutes on a cardio machine and be sure not to push yourself too hard. It will also be extra important to listen to your body and take a breather if you start to feel dizzy or light-headed which is going to happen much more often than it otherwise would.

If you ignore this advice and push your exercise intensity level to the limit then it will make the rest of your workout feel like much more of a struggle regardless of what you are doing.

2) Timing is everything

This is not to say that you are never going to want to push yourself while you are fasting, rather, it is just important to pick the right times to do so. The most productive time to take on an especially strenuous workout is going to about an hour after you have broken your fast. This will give your body enough time to fuel up and also ensure that you will be able to restock your reserves before your next fasting period as well.

3) Plan Your Meals Around Your Workouts

Health experts recommend working out on an empty stomach. This is a fantastic idea especially if your personal goal is to lose weight. Consider going for an early morning jog or a spin class. Even then, you need to eat the right kind of meals for dinner prior to working out. Basically, if you know that you are going to exercise, then you should consider what you are going to have for your meals the day before.

If you are planning a cardio workout in the morning, for instance, then you should build your glycogen stores with complex carbohydrates. If you have these for dinner the night before, then you will have sufficient energy for your workouts the following morning. You never want to workout on a full stomach. The important point to note is the need to plan ahead such that your nutrition needs to match the demands of your workouts even when you exercise early in the morning.

Best Approach to Working Out

You should exercise to your heart's content unless you start feeling lightheaded because of fasting. According to some elite athletes, strength tends to peak after a 16-hour or longer fasting period. You will soon realize that the more your body gets used to fasting, the easier the exercises get and the more benefits you'll gain.

Now if your main source of energy is based on a carb-centered diet, then you should be careful when doing intense exercises. This is because you may easily run out of fuel and start feeling weak, nauseous, lightheaded, and dizzy. Feeling weak and nauseous is likely to occur when your glycogen levels are depleted which is highly likely when you are fasting. However, if you opt for less intense workouts, then your body will start burning fat for energy. This is ideal for women seeking to lose weight and get rid of fat around the tummy.

If you are new to intermittent fasting, then you should not engage in any intense workouts, at least not at the beginning. This is because your blood sugar is likely to drop rapidly and you could start feeling dizzy. Therefore, always pay attention to your body as it will alert you on how far you can go and when the best time to stop is. Always remember, a little planning goes a long way so plan ahead and be prepared when it is time to workout.

Also, before working out, consider the length of your workouts. For instance, are you fasting for 8 hours on your fast day, or is it 12 hours? This will help determine what time your workouts should begin. The length of your fasting hours will also help determine which meals are most suitable for you.

Balancing Intermittent Fasting with Intense Workouts

The same applies to intermittent fasting lifestyle. You should ensure that you understand the nitty-gritty of each intermittent fasting protocol that you plan to try. If you are used to having breakfast each morning, then you will very likely feel weak and sluggish during your morning workouts. It is possible to feel this way when you first start out because your body is not yet used to nutrient deprivation.

This tends to happen to most people when they first start out so do not worry when it happens to you. Many beginners find it difficult to identify the right balance between proper workout and a suitable eating schedule. Fortunately, there is a lot of credible information from sports nutritionists and professional athletes on how to balance workouts and meals, even for beginners.

Feel free to adjust your exercise or eating schedule

Intermittent fasting need not feel like an absolutely strict way of living. This lifestyle actually offers you plenty of wiggle room, allowing you to set the rules that suit you. The aim is to find the ideal exercise and workout time. You can try and schedule your eating around your ideal workout schedule to fuel up adequately before and after a workout session.

Sports nutritionists suggest working out during your feeding window. If you workout during your feeding window, you will be able to have your meal immediately after an intense workout session. You will also be able to enjoy a healthy snack before your workouts. Think about exercises such as taking a brisk 20 to 30-minute walk in the park or around your neighborhood, which is not as intensive as the sweat sessions you may be used to. If you prefer working out in the morning, then you can reschedule your eating window to the 8.00 am - 4.00 pm window. This will shift your fasting hours so that you begin at 4.00 pm until the following morning.

Make your workouts more effective

An intermittent fasting lifestyle requires that you adopt new ideas, for instance, fasting equals losing. If your aim of starting this lifestyle is to lose weight, then working out should be an added bonus. Also, remember that when you fast, you burn fat, but it is your post workout nutrition that helps you develop strong, lean muscles.

If you want to lose weight, then you should pay closer attention to your nutrition and eating plans rather than your workout routine. This might come as a shocker due to your previous understanding of exercise, fasting, and dieting. Try and focus more on certain types of workouts over others to significantly lose weight. This will largely depend on what your body would allow on a given day.

Give intermittent fasting workouts time to settle in

Just like it is with everything else in your life, give your body time to accept intermittent fasting and workouts. We all have different bodies, and some will adjust faster than others. Some people are totally comfortable working out in a fasted state, for example. Most people often fast and work out hoping to see immediate results. This can result in frustration and a desire to give up. A lot of these people end up giving up simply because they did not give the lifestyle enough time to settle in. For some, it can take about two weeks only to adjust to intermittent fasting. Others often take longer depending on a number of circumstances.

Experts refer to different personal circumstances as clutter. Apparently, the focus is often to clear the clutter before doing anything else. For instance, you have to deal with issues such as your busy schedule, your stress levels, health challenges, deficiencies, and so much more. If the "clutter" is not cleared off at the onset, then you will not be able to come up with new habits, proper work out schedules, and things like that.

You must plan your meals

Timing is everything when it comes to intermittent fasting and working out. Even then, the quality of your meals is just as important. Sports nutritionists suggest making your final meal in your feeding window one that is capable of sustaining you well through the fasting period. This should be a meal of healthy fats, proteins, and non-starchy vegetables.

When you consume such a meal at the end of your feeding window, you will set yourself up to feel full and satisfied even as you begin the fasting period. On the other hand, consuming a meal that consists mostly of carbohydrates towards the end of your feeding window will only set you up for cravings and hunger during your fast period. Protein and fiber-rich meals will usually hold you over through the night and till the next feeding window.

Remember to stay motivated

It is important to stay motivated when you start intermittent fasting. You need to always remember where you are coming from and where it is you are going if you are to succeed. This works well in any sphere of your life including health and wellness. Consider all the reason that made you start fasting and what your goals are. You can even write these reasons down and state your goals. This way, you will be motivated to stay the course and watch your health and life transform right before you. People do not quit because they are tired or burned out, usually it is because they forgot the reason why they started in the first place

Cardio Exercises and Fasting

Exercising during fasting has been proven to have several fitness and health benefits. According to Dr. Joseph Mercola M.D., a health practitioner and researcher in Chicago, Illinois, the combination of cardio exercises and fasting leads to the breakdown of glycogen and fat for energy which stimulates the body to burn fat without affecting muscle. Many health experts are of the opinion that intermittent fasting and cardio workouts provide an effective way of losing weight.

There are different ways of doing intermittent fasting. For instance, you can cut back your calories if it makes your cardio workouts more efficient. This simply means consuming less food on your fast days for more effective workouts. However, on eating days, you can maintain your normal calorie count. If you are looking to cutting down your weight and losing stubborn fat around your tummy, then intermittent fasting and cardio exercises can help you achieve this.

According to health experts, intermittent fasting offers all the benefits of eating less but without the rigors of fasting regularly. This is because you enjoy eating normally on most days, but you still benefit. But there are ways to boost the health benefits of intermittent fasting and supercharge your weight loss. You do so by adding cardio exercises to your workout routines.

According to research scientists, if you combine intermittent fasting with cardio workouts, you are likely to lose a lot more weight with this arrangement compared to fasting but without cardio workouts. Studies show that the diet-and-exercise combination not only results in more weight loss but also helps your blood lipids. Blood lipids are a good indicator of heart or cardio risk. Participants in the study showed decreased LDL which is the "bad" cholesterol and an increase in HDL which is the beneficial cholesterol.

Health experts have always thought that a good diet is much more important in maintaining good body weight than exercise. However, from the above studies, it is now evident that a combination of cardio exercises and a good diet can go a long way in weight management than either approach alone.

Recommended cardio exercises with intermittent fasting for weight loss include;

- Cycling
- Running
- Jumping rope
- HIIT

High-intensity interval training involves short bursts of exercises done at close to maximum heart rate followed by brief recovery periods. It can also involve slightly longer bursts of cardio exercises at close to 90% of maximum heart rate. These intense training workouts are more effective than slow endurance training even though they take much less time.

Ideally, you can adapt an intermittent fasting plan with 500 calories on fasting and cardio workout days then eat normally on non-fasting days. You combine this with a high-intensity training program at 90 percent of maximum heart rate, and you will lose weight and become super-fit.

Therefore, if you wish to lose weight, then a combination of cardio and nutrition will serve you well. However, you need to make intermittent fasting a lifestyle that you can keep even after you lose weight. This way, you will maintain a healthy body and enjoy all other benefits brought on by the intermittent fast lifestyle

Weight Training and Intermittent Fasting

Ideally, you should do both cardio exercises and weights training. This is true both for your fast and non-fast days. A lot of it will depend on your long-term goals and preferences.

Experts advise both women and men to do cardio on their fasting days and weights training on non-fasting days.

Fasted Weight Training for Morning Session

The main concern during fasted weight training is whether or not to have a post-workout meal or snack. This fact is especially true on fasting days. However, what is of ultimate importance is your total calorie consumption for the entire day. You really need to structure your diet such that it is as tasty and enjoyable as possible.

If you choose to workout on your fasting day, then you should push your first meal to the afternoon. This way, you will be able to workout during the morning session then have lunch later in the afternoon. Let's assume you wake up at 7.00 am in the morning, you will need to take a simple pre-workout supplement. This is not mandatory but optional. You should then workout between 7.30 am, and 8.30 am. After you finish your workout, take a shower and rest until 12.00 noon. Have a fruit such as an apple then your first meal at 2.00 pm.

One of the key protocols of successful weightlifting routines is to keep your training sessions as focused and intense as possible. Think of strategies such as the reverse pyramid. This is a training strategy for muscle gain and massive strength. This type of strategy requires that you start with the heaviest set first. It means doing the heaviest work when you are still fresh and fully capable. With each set, you become fatigued with lower energy levels. The best part of this strategy is that you can give your all in the first set knowing that you won't need to replicate it again. This makes it so easy to progress.

Go to the Gym Prepared

If you are using fasted weight training while pushing for personal records and training hard 3 times a week, then you will surely build an impressive physique. Intermittent fasting will make it easy for you to build strong muscle while staying lean. However, you will need to consume sufficient protein levels to build strong, lean muscle.

Always go to the gym with a plan or workout regime. You should also record your workouts to enable you to keep track of your progress and workout plan. This provides you with the ability to improve and get better. Lastly, remember to stay focused and stick not just with the workout plan but the entire intermittent fasting lifestyle.

Ensure After-workout Meals are Nutritious

It is advisable to save more of your calorie and food consumption for the evening regardless of when you train. Instead of worrying about post-workout snacks or meals, it is better to consider having a meal that you will enjoy and one that is nutritious and will replenish the energy spent. If you stick to your meal schedule, then pre and post workout snacks are really not that important.

Track Your Workouts

Even as you lift weights and workout on a regular basis, you should track your progress. If you work hard and remain consistent, then you will watch your physique transform. If you are making weekly progress with your fasting workout routine, then you should be able to lift heavier weights progressively as time goes by.

Weights training can be done two to three times each week. You can do weights training on your fast days and aerobics training on your non-fast days. If this works well for you, then you should stick to this training routine. The bottom line is that you are comfortable, happy, and seeing progress. If something makes you uncomfortable or if the schedule isn't quite working out for you, then you can consider changing your schedule.

Chapter 8: Common Mistakes & Tips

Anyone who practices intermittent fasting as a lifestyle is bound to experience tremendous benefits including better sleep, increased mental clarity and ability to better manage food cravings. Many attest to the health benefits and general wellbeing after weeks of practicing this lifestyle.

However, these benefits can only be realized if this lifestyle is practiced correctly. Sadly, people make mistakes and end up losing out on some or all of these benefits. For instance, some try to do too much within a short time period while others give up too soon.

By avoiding these common mistakes and applying this healthy lifestyle correctly, you will be successful and will realize the benefits of intermittent fasting a lot sooner than you think.

Common Mistakes with Intermittent Fasting

There are plenty of people who get the basics of this lifestyle the first time around. This is all well and good. However, this is not always the case and some women still get a few things wrong. Here is a look at some of the common mistakes that people often make and how to avoid them.

Choosing the wrong fasting protocol

There are different fasting protocols allowed so finding the right one is crucial. When determining the right kind of protocol, you need to consider your lifestyle. For instance, how busy is your lifestyle? If you have a demanding occupation, then you may want to find the right protocol for you. Therefore, check out the different intermittent fasting protocols and identify the one that best suits your lifestyle.

Not consuming enough fat

It is important to consume sufficient amounts of fat with your meals. Fat helps prevent the ups and downs of reactive hypoglycemia and sustains your blood sugar. When you do not take enough fat, your insulin goes up, and blood sugar plays up. Then your blood sugar levels drop, and adrenals have to push it back up. This is not a desirable situation at all. Fortunately, good quality, healthy fat can help manage this situation. This is fat sourced from coconut oil or avocado.

Unresolved hormonal issues:

If you have high blood sugar levels, thyroid problems, female hormones imbalance, or adrenal glands challenges, then you shouldn't be cutting out those meals just yet. This is because your body is already suffering a physiology problem. If your body is not nourished early morning and early afternoon, then your body may be stressed out. You should first consider getting these issues sorted out first by health practitioner then seek advice about leading an intermittent fasting lifestyle.

Not consuming sufficient calories

Fasting tends to affect the hormones that regulate hunger such that you won't feel as hungry. This way, you are likely to consume very little food. You need to be very careful not to consume too few calories because your body will be deprived of essential nutrition. You should eat at least 1200 calories as a minimum. If you do not do this then you will feel extremely hungry the following day and this could affect your ability to perform.

You are scared of feeling hungry

Many people get scared of feeling hungry in the course of the day due to fasting. Yet we all feel hungry at some point during the day even if we consume six meals per day. The problem with this kind of issue is that people often want to eat the minute they feel hungry. The truth is that your body is capable of going without a meal for lengthy periods of time, even 24 hours.

You consume too much junk food

Intermittent fasting is never about what you eat but when you eat. While this is a good mantra to abide with, it sometimes results in problems due to the foods we eat. Most people actually do not know what to eat. Yet it is possible to consume sumptuous meals that are healthy and good for you. Your focus should be more on animal and plant products, both of which should be unprocessed. While this sounds like a paleo diet, it simply refers to having any and all meats and fish. Also, eat foods that grow in the garden such as vegetables, fruits, grains, and pulses and much more. You can consume some processed foods as well. However, try and eat mostly natural foods.

You do not lead an active lifestyle

It is very important to stay busy throughout your fasting period. If you are not busy, then you tend to feel hungry and want to eat anything and everything on site. It is important, especially when starting out, to always keep busy and avoid sitting idle. You can try and schedule something so that you are not around food. Basically, if food is not around, then you will not be tempted. Avoid places with free donuts or where you have friends having meals or snacks.

Abusing stimulants

It is not uncommon for people to take too much coffee. This is wrong because you can end up with a caffeinated euphoria. It is okay to have one or two cups to kick-start your fast day. What you need to avoid is becoming over-reliant on coffee to get through the day. If you have to, drink a cup or two and leave it at that. Try not to consume more coffee after your lunch break.

You start off way too ambitious

All too often, people start a diet program or a healthy lifestyle like intermittent fasting with high expectations. It takes most people a long time to get used to hunger and coping with it. You should not be too hard on yourself and do not be way too ambitious. Going from regular eating to a single meal per day can come as quite a shock to most people. Go easy on yourself and cut yourself some slack. You should not try to achieve everything all at once but instead, try and take one step at a time.

You think that more is better

Sometimes people tend to think that fasting for longer means better outcomes and better results. This is not necessarily the case. While intermittent fasting for 16 hours per day is recommended, you should not fast beyond 20 to 24 hours. You will do more harm than good if you increase your fasting hours unnecessarily. In fact, according to a recent study, most fasting benefits begin to dwindle past the 20-hour mark.

Being obsessed with time

Some people are obsessed with time and cannot be flexible. You need to embrace a relaxed lifestyle without undue concern about hours, seconds, and minutes. Basically, an obsessed person stares at the clock and thinks that a single minute past time will ruin their entire fast experience. Many experienced people will eat anytime within their eating window without worrying about the minutes or seconds. If you freed yourself from the 6-meals-a-day program, then you should free yourself from the clock.

Some tend to give up too soon:

Intermittent fasting is a lifestyle that requires a certain amount of discipline. It also takes a bit of time to get used to. Health and nutrition experts know that the initial four to five days are the most challenging. You can expect to feel, exhausted, lightheaded, and hungry. The best part is that these feelings will pass quickly and by the end of the first week, the body will begin to adapt. You will begin to feel more focused, energetic, and the hunger will diminish and eventually disappear. Therefore, rather than giving up too soon, assess your situation after the first week and see if you can make any adjustments.

Working out excessively

If you are physically unfit and are just starting out with intermittent fasting, then be very careful not to do anything excessively, especially exercising. The best approach to exercising is to ease yourself into a routine. In fact, both fasting and exercising require a gradual approach. It would be disastrous as a beginner to join a 5-day intense workout program. Your body is already trying to adjust to limited food intake so an intense workout can lead to fatigue and possibly hospitalization. A little bit of physical strain every now and then is good for the body but too much all at once can be a problem.

How to Fight Hunger Pangs

1. **Have the right mindset when it comes to intermittent fasting:** The first thing we need to note is that you will not suffer serious setbacks due to fasting. If you are just an hour into a fast and you start feeling hungry, convincing yourself that this is not possible, and begin obsessing over your next meal, then this will not work. Instead, focus on reasons why you decided to fast and about the benefits it affords your body.

2. **Learn to discern between physical and psychological hunger:** There is a huge difference between physical and psychological or emotional hunger. Physical hunger can be satisfied with any type of food. It comes gradually and can be postponed, causes satisfaction without guilt, and you stop eating once you feel full. This contradicts emotional hunger which comes suddenly and feels rather urgent. Psychological hunger causes specific cravings and causes you to eat more than you should. It causes you to feel uncomfortably fill and leaves you feeling guilty and mad at your actions.

3. **Keep your mind and body active:** Try and keep busy, especially on your fasting days. Try and find something enjoyable to do. Basically, you need to immerse yourself into activities that you enjoy, especially in the morning period. This is when you are most productive. When you are busy and in a state of flow, time flies very fast. Even as you remain active, you will be burning fats and also losing weight.

4. ***Try one or two tablespoons of Psyllium Husk:*** Psyllium Husk is an edible, soluble fiber with immense benefits to your body. It is also prebiotic and is often given as a dietary supplement. When you take this product, it will expand and draw water from your colon. It sweeps waste out of the colon efficiently and eliminates it. You will not feel bloated or full if you take this product during your fasting period. In addition, Psyllium is also known to positively affect cholesterol levels and promotes a healthy heart.

5. **Hunger during fasting**: As you begin your intermittent fasting journey, you will soon learn that hunger is only an issue in the initial stages. Once your body starts getting used to the lifestyle, you will find it easier to cope. You are likely to suffer hunger only the first 2 to 3 weeks. After the fourth week, hunger should not really be a major issue.

Chapter 9: Staying Motivated

Make Intermittent Fasting Easier on your Body

1. Take Beverages and Water to Stay Hydrated

This tip is basically the easiest of them all yet it is one of the most avoided. You need to drink a lot of water and other beverages throughout the day. Not everyone loves the taste of water or having to go to the bathroom every half an hour. Nevertheless, it is crucial to ensure that you are drinking as close to a gallon of water per day as possible because being in a fasted state will cause your body to become dehydrated faster than would otherwise be the case. What's more, drinking more water will actually cause you to feel more full, more regularly, making the fasting process easier as a result.

Even then, taking water frequently has its numerous benefits. One of these is to keep you satisfied, so you do not feel hungry most of the time. A lot of the time, the hunger we feel is often dehydration. It is therefore important that you drink lots of water and stay hydrated throughout the day.

Apart from water, you can also have a cup of tea or coffee. Even then, to remain hydrated, take water throughout the day. When you are without food in your system, the body takes the opportunity to detoxify the liver. The water you drink will be used to clear out the toxins. If you do not drink water, the toxins will be eliminated with reserve water in your body. This will leave you quite dehydrated.

Your body also benefits immensely when you drink water. If you are dehydrated, you will not be able to workout energetically or at peak levels. To be successful at intermittent fasting, remember to drink plenty of water throughout the day.

2. Drink Bone Broth

Alternatively, you can drink bone broth when you are fasting. If you get bored of water and other beverages, then give bone broth a try. You can choose to prepare some at home or buy pre-packed at the local grocery store.

Broth contains very little calories which is negligible in our case. However, the benefits of the micronutrients in bone broth are immense. For many years, this broth has been acknowledged as an effective appetite suppressant. Studies confirm that it actually can suppress appetite in mammals. It is thought to have anti-obesity properties and is well known for regulating blood sugar.

Should hunger pangs persist as you fast, then heat one cup and consume. One cup is sufficient to suppress hunger and keep you satiated until time for your meal.

3. **Consider enlisting professional support:**

You should consult a health expert before fully embarking on this very beneficial lifestyle. A health expert can guide you through the changes you need to make and enable you to transition safely into the intermittent fasting lifestyle. You should consider seeking advice instead of trying to guess what is right for you.

How to Stay Motivated as You Fast

Most people start off any diet really motivated at the beginning but then get discouraged when they do not get the results they want fast enough. First, you need to understand that this is a lifestyle and not an overnight diet. You also need to understand that nothing is easy or instant. Everything takes a little time. Here are some tips that can help you stay motivated.

Use a mirror and not the scales

At the start of your diet, take a look at yourself after a shower. Observe your body closely and notice which parts need toning and where you need to lose some fat. You can also take a picture of yourself and keep observing changes on a regular basis. Avoid using a weighing scale because it is bound to discourage you.

Eat a variety of foods

Nobody enjoys eating the same food each day. You need to find out which are the best foods possible for fasting days and ensure to eat healthy on your free days. Once you get to discover great foods, you will be able to discover new recipes and how to prepare meals that you actually enjoy.

Start with a friend

When you start the intermittent fasting lifestyle, find someone you can partner with. It could be a partner, family member, spouse, or a close friend. Go through the diet with him/her and use each other as a coach when working out. You can also motivate and cheer each other up. Having someone to plan meals with and go grocery shopping with is a great way to stay motivated.

Even as you fast, remember to continue maintaining a healthy lifestyle. Learn to eat healthy foods and have a balanced diet always. Always choose fresh produce and unprocessed foods. If you get enough rest each day, workout regularly, and fast periodically, then you will soon be healthier, look better, lose weight, and enjoy all the benefits that come with intermittent fasting.

Check out other Books by Jamie Connor

<u>Meal Prep – Ultimate Guide</u>

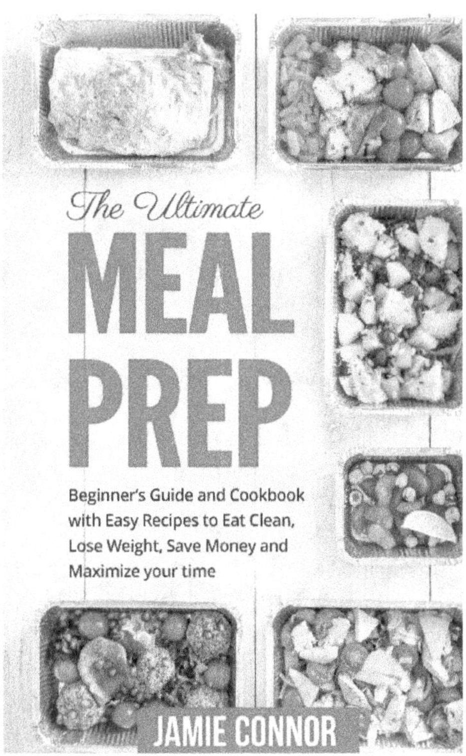

One Final Thing…

Did You Enjoy and Find This Book Useful?

If you did, please let me know by leaving a review on AMAZON. Reviews lets Amazon knows that I am providing quality material to my readers. Even a few words and rating would go a long way. I would like to thank you in advance for your time.

If you didn't, please shoot me an email at jamieconnor@bmccpublishing.com and let me know what you didn't like. I maybe able to change or update it.

Lastly, if you have any feedback to improve the book, please email me. In this age, this book can be a living book. It can be continuously improved by feedback provided by readers like you.

About The Author

Jamie Connor is a certified personal trainer, yoga instructor, and nutrition coach that currently lives in Miami Florida. After graduating from Cornell University with a Ms in Nutrition, Jamie is currently working for a Fortune 500 company in Miami. Growing up in a family that consumed a lot of process foods, Jamie struggled with obesity and health problems. After almost losing her life 6 years ago, Jamie made a decision to develop a healthy lifestyle. When Jamie started exercising and eliminating processed foods from her diet, things started to turn around. She felt stronger and energy levels were through the roof.

Today, Jamie is on a mission to share what she had learned with her readers to get the same results. In addition, through multiple trial and errors, she developed many healthy and delicious recipes that are full of flavor, texture and wholesome nutrition.

Jamie also enjoys practicing yoga, reading, and traveling around the world to discover new recipes.